# Obesity Antidote In Modern world; The Ultimate Antidote For Weight Loss And Medication

Jamie P.Louis

Thank you for selecting "OBESITY ANTIDOTE IN MODERN WORLD." It offers easy measures on" Obesity "in today's world.

You can also get more interesting books of Jamie Louis like:

OBESITY CODE AND MANAGEMENT

METHOD TO PARENTING TEENS

# Table of contents

# Table of contents

# Chapter 1

Understanding Modern Day's Obesity

Obesity was dubbed "the pediatric pandemic of the new millennium" by the American Academy of Pediatrics in 2005. Children who are overweight or obese are increasingly being diagnosed with type II diabetes, high blood pressure, and increased cholesterol. was nearly entirely observed in adults. In addition, children who are overweight are more likely than children who are of normal weight to suffer from fractured bones and joint issues. Pediatricians and public health professionals are very concerned about the long-term effects of childhood obesity since obese children are at a greater risk of becoming fat adults. If the growing rate of obesity is not stopped, longevity experts have determined that today's American youngsters may "live less healthy and probably even shorter lives than their parents."

Additionally, efforts were being made to create more effective techniques for preventing childhood obesity, such as those that may foretell a baby's future propensity for being overweight or obese. One such tool, which was reported in 2012, was found to be able to accurately predict the risk of newborn obesity by taking into account the newborn's weight, the maternal and paternal BMIs, the number of people living in the household with the newborn, the occupation of the mother, and the mother's smoking habits during pregnancy.

reasons for obesity

Find out how the leptin protein was discovered in mice and how it may be used to treat diabetes and obesity in people.
Find out how the leptin protein was discoverec in mice and how it may be used to treat diabetes and obesity in people.
all videos related to this post
Hear how research on uncommon ailments like lipodystrophy aids in understanding the genetic mechanisms of diabetes and obesity.
Hear how research on uncommon ailments like lipodystrophy aids in understanding the genetic mechanisms of diabetes and obesity.
all videos related to this post
Genome-wide association studies have discovered genetic differences in small numbers of people with morbid obesity, whether it be adult or childhood-onset, among European and other Caucasian groups. In one study, a subpopulation of highly obese people with childhood-onset obesity had a chromosomal loss implicating 30 genes. Less than 1% of the morbidly obese research participants had the deleted region, but its absence was thought to lead to abnormal hormone signaling, namely of leptin and insulin, which control hunger and glucose metabolism, respectively.

Hyperphagia, overeating, and tissue insulin resistance are linked to hormonal dysregulation, which raises the risk of type II diabetes. Morbid obesity may have a hereditary component, at least in some cases, as evidenced by the discovery of chromosomal abnormalities in afflicted people.

The reasons for obesity, however, are more complicated for the majority of those who are afflicted and include the interaction of several variables. Indeed, rather than a dramatic change in human genetics, the fast rise in obesity throughout the world is likely caused by considerable changes in environmental variables and behavioral changes. For instance, early eating habits imposed by an obese mother on her kids may have a significant impact on the cultural transmission of obesity from one generation to the next as opposed to genetic transmission. Similarly, links between childhood obesity and procedures like cesarean sections, whose prevalence has significantly increased globally, suggest that environment and behavior may have a more significant impact on the early beginnings of obesity than previously believed. More broadly, a nation's particular way of life and each person's behavioral and emotional response to it may have a substantial role in the prevalence of obesity. In wealthy communities, an abundance of readily available high-calorie foods and drinks, along with more sedentary lifestyle choices that significantly lower calorie requirements, can easily result in overeating. Some people resort to food and alcoholic beverages for "relief" from the worries and anxieties of contemporary life. Researchers have discovered that diets high in sugars and saturated fats, lack of exercise, and the accessibility of cheap processed foods are the main causes of obesity in every nation.

Children become fat when they eat too much and move too little, even if the underlying reasons for juvenile obesity are complicated and not entirely understood. Additionally, a lot of kids make poor eating choices, favoring unhealthy, sugary snacks over nutritious fruits and vegetables. Lack of calorie-burning activity has also been a significant factor in the rise of childhood obesity. According to a 2005 poll, American children between the ages of 8 and 18 watched television and movies for an average of four hours each day, and they also spent an extra two hours using computers and playing video games. Additionally, consuming too much fat when pregnant by the mother encourages children to overeat. Children, for instance, tend to appreciate fatty foods more if their moms consumed a high-fat diet when they were pregnant. The prenatal brain's alterations brought on by fat appear to be the physiological foundation for this. For instance, brain cells in growing fetuses of pregnant rats fed high-fat diets create a substantial amount of appetite-stimulating proteins known as orexigenic peptides. Following delivery and for the duration of the child's life, these peptides are still generated in large amounts. In contrast to rats whose mothers ingested normal quantities of lipids throughout pregnancy, these rats eat more, weigh more, and reach sexual maturity earlier in life.

Obesity's consequences on health

Obesity is a major medical issue in addition to being unattractive, especially in regions of the world where being thin is the preferred appearance. Obese people often have shorter life expectancies and experience several diseases early, more frequently, and more severely than people of normal weight. For instance, fat individuals usually get diabetes; in fact, type II diabetes accounts for around 90% of cases globally. In addition to being a substantial risk factor for cancer, obesity accounts for one in every twenty-five cases of cancer diagnosed globally as of 2018. Researchers discovered that among relatively young individuals between the ages of 25 and 49 in the United States, the prevalence of cancer linked to obesity was rising.

Obese people are at risk for experiencing an accelerated rate of cognitive decline as they age due to the link between obesity and the worsening of cardiovascular health, which appears in diseases like diabetes and hypertension (abnormally high blood pressure). Increased body fat is linked to the atrophy (withering away) of brain tissue, notably in the temporal and frontal lobes of the brain, according to studies on brain size in people with long-term obesity. In reality, a BMI of 25 or above, which includes both obesity and overweight, is linked to shrinkage of the brain, which raises the chance of dementia, the most prevalent type of which is Alzheimer's disease.

Obese women frequently struggle with infertility, take longer to conceive than women of normal weight and have a higher chance of miscarriage when they become pregnant. Since extra body fat is linked to lower testosterone levels, obese men are also more likely to experience reproductive issues. Obese people general y have a higher chance of acquiring cancer and dying young from degenerative illnesses of the heart, arteries, and kidneys compared to people of normal weight. Obese people have poor surgical risks and have a higher chance of accident-related mortality. Mental health is impacted; behavioral effects of an obese look, such as shyness and isolation as well as excessive self-assertion, may have neurotic or psychotic roots.

A well-known global pandemic that is affecting people everywhere is obesity. Obesity and its associated co-morbidities have been on the rise since the 1980s, despite several initiatives and recommendations to the contrary. The underlying causes of obesity have been discovered, and they are mostly related to a genetic susceptibility to gain weight from increased calorie intake and decreased energy expenditures, as well as a tendency to do so in the environment.

In addition, several structural environmental changes during the 1980s have created an obesogenic atmosphere characterized by the accessibility of high-calorie, poor-quality food and insufficient physical activity. All of this causes body weight to grow, contributing to a problem with global public health as well as a specific patient's illness that frequently does not improve with diets and exercise.

Fried food consumption needs to be limited in those who are genetically susceptible to obesity because it may interact with genes involved in fat metabolism.

Since many people who have these so-called "obesity genes" do not become overweight, healthy lives can lessen the effects of them. The impact of genes and gene-environment interactions on the development of obesity is briefly covered in this article.

In the twenty-first century, obesity is a health problem that impacts both wealthy and poor, educated and illiterate, Westernized and non-Westernized countries. The earliest obesity-related gene variants are found in the so-called "fat mass and obesity-associated" (FTO) gene on chromosome 16. The risk of obesity is 20–30% higher for people who have one of these highly common gene variants than for those who do not. Researchers identified the second obesity-related gene variant on chromosome 18, close to the melanocortin-4 receptor gene (the same gene responsible for a rare form of monogenic obesity).

It takes a very long time for new mutations or polymorphisms to spread. If our genes have virtually remained the same over the past 40 years despite rising obesity rates, what has changed? Our surroundings, which are made up of the social, political, economic, and physical elements that have an impact on our daily activities and eating patterns. Environmental factors that make it easier for individuals to overeat and harder for them to get enough exercise are largely to blame for the present rise in overweight and obesity.

The relationship between genes and environment and how it affects obesity is continually developing. My current study indicates that possessing so-called "obesity genes" does not typically result in getting overweight. Instead, it seems that adopting a balanced diet and engaging in regular exercise may help to mitigate some of the genetically predisposed risk of obesity. The majority of people probably have some genetic vulnerability to obesity depending on their family history and ethnicity. To transition from an inherited vulnerability to obesity itself, changes in nutrition, lifestyle, or other environmental factors are frequently required. These are only a handful of the changes.

The earliest obesity-related gene variants are found on chromosome 16, specifically in the "fat mass and obesity-associated" (FTO) gene. These gene variants are highly prevalent, and people who have one have a 20–30% higher risk of obesity than those who do not. The second obesity-related gene variant has been identified on chromosome 18, close to the melanocortin-4 receptor gene (the same gene responsible for a rare form of monogenic obesity).

The study of the interactions between genes and environments that influence obesity is still in its infancy. So-called "obesity genes" do not, in most circumstances, invariably result in being overweight, suggests studies to date. Instead, it seems that adopting a balanced diet and engaging in regular exercise may help to mitigate some of the genetically predisposed risk of obesity.

The majority of people probably have some genetic vulnerability to obesity depending on their family history and ethnicity. To transition from an inherited vulnerability to obesity itself, changes in nutrition, lifestyle, or other environmental factors are frequently required. Among the changes are the following:

food is now readily available at all times of day and in places that did not previously offer it, such as gas stations, pharmacies, and office supply stores; the proliferation of highly processed foods, fast food, and beverages with added sugars; a sharp decline in physical activity during work, household tasks, and free time, especially among kids; an increase in the amount of time spent watching television, using computers, and partaking in other sedentary activities.

Human development, physiology, and adaption are all impacted by genes. Everyone is susceptible to fat. Surprisingly little is known, however, about the particular genes that contribute to obesity as well as the extent of so-called "genetic environment interactions," or the complex relationships between our history and upbringing.

Chapter 2

Energy, A new Eating Plan, And Workout

Breakfast, lunch, and dinner are the best times to eat if
you want to lose weight.
The time you decide to eat might be quite significant for
weight reduction.
Since weight loss advice typically focuses so heavily on
what to eat to lose weight, many of us neglect to take
other factors Into I account, such as the best time to eat
breakfast, lunch, and dinner.

Breakfast should be consumed as soon as possible in
the morning, ideally about 7:11 a.m. Additionally, rather
than later, it's recommended to consume your lunch
between 12.30 and 1 pm. The timing is ideal at 12:38.
Additionally, the worse it can be for your diet, the later
you have dinner. The study indicated that the optimal
time to eat dinner was around 6.14 p.m., so try to eat
between 6 and 6.30 p.m. It controls our hunger
hormones and keeps us fuller and happy for a longer .m
of time, but if you wake up later than usual and can't
envision making a healthy meal before the sun rises, it
is still beneficial.

your time for eating is "a matter of balance. To maintain
energy, it makes sensible to spread out your food
consumption throughout the remaining meals of the day.
Since our bodies strongly respond to the pattern, aim to
stick to a 1 p.m. luncheon and a 6 p.m. dinnertime if

your schedule allows it. Delaying meals until the late afternoon or evening might result in overeating or making bad nutritional choices."

When is the best time of day to snack?
Snacks are best consumed during 11.01 am, 3.14 pm, and 9.31 pm. You are most susceptible to lose your willpower at this stage. You should consider having a snack if you spend more than four hours between meals or just after a challenging exercise.

It's important to choose intelligently since not all of your go-to snacks will satisfy you in between meals. To help you feel satisfied for longer, choose meals that are strong in fiber and protein. It's important to always eat consciously, even while snacking. Keep your senses sharp and present. Plan your meals and healthy snacks in advance to help you choose and stick to healthier dietary habits. While eating a high-protein diet may be the best option in some situations, it's crucial to pay attention to how much protein you take in while attempting to feel satisfied. The author suggests against having too much protein at once, particularly if it is mixed with little or no fiber. There is always a limit to how much our body can absorb, therefore any surplus is made available to our gut microbes. Even while our gut microbes like high-fiber meals, if any undigested protein is consumed, they will start to breakdown it. Products from this process might be detrimental to lifespan and digestive health.

Which rule is most important when attempting to reduce weight?

The most important thing to remember is that you must consume less calories each day than you expend if you want to lose weight. Sadly, there is no other way to reduce weight. It may be done in a number of ways and is known as an energy deficit or calorie deficit. You won't see any benefits unless you're in this deficit, despite the fact that low-carb, high-fat regimens like the Banting diet and the 16:8 plan may sell themselves as definite methods to lose weight.
This is because when you eat, your body turns the nutrients in the food into energy. This energy is required by the organism for everything from breathing to movement. You will have excess energy if you eat more calories than your body needs; this energy will eventually be stored as fat. If you eat less than you need, you won't have enough energy, and your body will start using its fat stores for fuel. The last phase results in weight reduction.

What harm does skipping meals cause?
Under no circumstances should you miss meals.
It has been demonstrated that missing breakfast is associated with several unfavorable symptoms, such as weight gain and a changed glucose metabolism. Many claim that eating breakfast helps set the tone for a balanced diet throughout the day and decreases impulsive munching. By eating a well-balanced breakfast that contains high-fiber foods like berries and

a sufficient amount of protein, such as Greek yogurt, you may be able to boost your metabolism for the day.

Aerial view of a gray rural table with a mango-banana smoothie bowl, natural greek yogurt, chia seeds, and a honey-topped vegetarian dessert (Mango banana smoothie bowl with natural greek yogurt  and chia seeds)

But people don't only like skipping breakfast. With up to 57% of respondents skipping supper, it was the second most common meal to skip. In addition to weight increase, those who skipped lunch or dinner were more likely to be overweight. Women and men who skipped their final meal of the day were more likely to have chronic tiredness because they had less sleep at night. They were also more prone to smoke or engage in heavy drinking.

In addition to eating breakfast, lunch, and dinner at the suggested times, you should create a calorie deficit. To find out what yours are, glance at a calorie counter. You will learn your maintenance level and shortfall threshold from this. For instance, your daily calorie target to lose 0.25 kilos per week will be 1,677 calories if you're a 30-year-old woman who is 5 feet 4 inches tall and weighs 70 kilograms (the typical weight for persons in the UK).

Your day may look like this if you pass that line:

Breakfast
Try to consume 400 calories with one of these
low-calorie breakfast meals, if you can.

The blackcurrant bircher muesli has 395 calories.
A 250 ml glass of orange juice has 118 calories and a
fast farmhouse fry-up has 221 calories.
Compared to a tall coffee from Starbucks, which has 90
calories, Slimming World's smoked salmon muffins
contain 295 calories.

Limit your lunch to no more than 500 calories (between
12:30 and 1 pm). You'll need a boost around midday, so
it's crucial to give your body the nutrients and protein it
needs. For this, choose complex carbohydrates rather
than refined ones like those found in white bread, rice,
and pasta. After lunch, you won't feel run down and
you'll remain satisfied for longer.
Ainsley Harriott's chicken spaghetti with peas contains
426 calories.
390 calories in a tortilla with spring veggies
A fast Quorn lunch bowl and 1 wholemeal bun contain
155 calories altogether.

Dinner About 500 calories should be in the evening
meal, which should be consumed between 6 and 6.30
p.m. If you don't want to feel too full before bed, it's best
to focus your meal on protein and vegetables rather
than choosing a spaghetti dish that is high in
carbohydrates.
mildly spiced chicken and chickpeas: 309 energy

A split pea and vegetable curry has 300 calories, while peppers and spicy turkey stuffing have 302 calories. Eat no more than 400, 500, and 500 calories for breakfast, lunch, and dinner, respectively. If you succeed, you can treat yourself to two 100-calorie snacks during the day. You will consume an additional 77 calories if you add milk to your tea or coffee.

There isn't a secret medication that can instantly shed pounds, and losing weight is harder said than done. As an alternative, you must consume fewer calories than you expend. This calls for a balanced diet, as well as cardio and weight exercise.

Ready to lose those extra pounds? Here are some of the top aerobic and strength-training activities for losing weight, along with advice on how to stay active all day.

4 aerobic workouts to lose weight

Your heart rate increases during cardiovascular exercises (or simply "cardio"). These are some of the best exercises for weight reduction because, according to Multazim Shaikh, a fitness expert and nutritionist with FamFits, the faster your heartbeat, the more fat you'll burn.

According to the Mayo Clinic, you need up to 300 minutes of moderate physical exercise each week to lose weight or keep it off. This takes place five days a week on average for 60 minutes.

Divide your cardio into three short exercises a day if you're busy. As an illustration, you might walk for 20 minutes during your lunch break, exercise for 20 minutes before bed, and repeat.

Excellent cardiac exercises to aid with weight loss include:

1. low-impact cardio
You can lose weight without engaging in vigorous activity. Low-intensity exercise can also help you burn calories and lose weight if you're a novice or have physical limitations.

Jogging, biking, power walking, swimming, and aerobics are some of the exercises on this list. As you become used to your new regimen, start slowly and gradually increase the intensity.

Five days a week, aim for 60 minutes of low-intensity cardio. Carry hand weights when jogging, strolling, or doing aerobics as your physical fitness improves.

2. Jog a rope
According to Shaikh, jumping rope not only enhances your ability to coordinate and think clearly but also raises your heart rate and helps you burn roughly 1,300 calories every hour.

Jump for 8 to 10 reps to warm up.

After that, leap without stopping for 1.5 minutes.
Repeat after a 15–30 second break.
Finish three sets.
You can alter your regimen as well. Jump one set while standing still, one set while using both legs, and one set while using just one leg.

3. Burpees
Squats, leaps, and pushups are combined into burpees. According to Shaikh, the workout is successful because you work out several muscle groups, including your chest, legs, and core, and you burn fat from your whole body.

30 seconds of 10 repetitions followed by 30 seconds of break.
Repeat five times.

4. Training with High-Intensity Intervals (HIIT)
Due to its potential to boost fat reduction and calorie burn, this cardio exercise has become more and more popular. It entails short bursts of vigorous activity that raise your heart rate, followed by a 15-second rest period.

If you don't have a lot of time, HIIT is fantastic. You may work out for a shorter period while still getting into a more challenging and demanding workout. You'll thus continue to burn calories for hours after your workout, according to Shaikh.

Here is an illustration of a HIIT workout:

Kicks the butt for 45 seconds, followed by a 15-second break.
Next, do 45 seconds of leaping lunges, then 15 seconds of rest.
Burpees for 45 seconds, followed by 15 seconds of rest.
Repeat ten to twenty times.
Incorporate additional exercises like jump squats and mountain climbers.
Alternatively, you might try performing a HIIT exercise on a treadmill:

For five minutes, warm up.
After that, sprint for a full minute at a high rate of speed.
After 30 seconds of walking, run for a minute at a high rate of speed.
Finish eight to ten sets.
5 weight-loss workouts that build strength
Don't overlook weight training or strength training when trying to lose weight, even though strength training alone doesn't produce quick results.

These workouts help rev up your metabolism. According to Stephanie Blozy, an expert in exercise science and owner of Fleet Feet in West Hartford, Connecticut, you will burn more calories both while exercising and at rest because they help you develop lean muscle mass.

Excellent weightlifting and strength-training routines to aid in weight loss include:

1. swinging a kettlebell
According to Boozy, this strenuous, all-over workout will raise your heart rate while boosting your arm and leg strength and assisting in the development of a strong core.

Swing a kettlebell with two hands for 20 seconds.
Take 8 seconds to relax.
8 times total.
Boozy advise lifting heavier weights more quickly to increase your heart rate and complete a cardio-intensive workout.

2. Pushups
Pushups are a great workout for strengthening your upper body, stabilizing your core, and adding muscle to your arms.

Beginners should begin with three sets of 10 repetitions, with a 60- to 90-second break in between each set. As your strength increases, gradually up the number of repetitions.

3. Lunges
Because you can perform lunges forward, backward, with weight or without weight, Blozy explains, "I enjoy the alternatives lunges bring." Hold a kettlebell or weight plate next to your chest for the weighted variant, or hoist the weight above for an even greater challenge.

Perform 1 set of 8–12 lunges on each leg.

## 4. Step-ups

Step-ups are another excellent workout that Blozy suggests doing to strengthen your legs while also stabilizing your core and lower back muscles. Start with a low step height (6 to 12 inches) and work your way up to something higher (like 24 to 30 inches).

Perform 5 sets of 5–10 repetitions on each side.
Do you want to make things difficult? According to Boozy, you may add weight by holding a dumbbell or kettlebell close to your chest or in each hand. You'll sweat profusely, your pulse rate will increase, and your quadriceps will burn.

## 5. Deadlifts

Boozy also offers deadlifts as a workout to tone your upper and lower body while losing weight. To make it seem more like cardio than weight training, she advises lowering the load to 50 to 70 percent of your maximum and increasing the reps.

Complete 1–3 sets of 10–20 repetitions.
PHYSICAL SOLUTIONS

Are you looking for further advice on health issues? Get in touch with services and assets that can assist you in achieving your health objectives.

Tell us what's currently affecting your health:

Easy methods to stay active each day
Look for other methods to stay active each day in addition to a regular exercise regimen and a nutritious diet.

Keep in mind that you'll burn more calories the more you exercise. This will enable you to lose the most weight possible and move closer to your objective.

While on the phone, during the show's commercial breaks, or in between episodes, pace the room.
Instead of using the elevator, use the stairs.
Cars should be parked in the back of garages.
Purchase a fitness tracker. Some activity monitors inform you when you've been inactive for too long. These notifications prompt you to move.
Make plans to go on walks with your employees.
Sit in your seat and fidget by tapping your hand, swinging your knee, or contracting your abs. Fidgeting may result in an additional 350 calories being burned each day for obese persons, claims one study trusted Source.
Take the bus or metro one stop sooner and continue walking the remaining distance to your destination.
While preparing meals or performing other domestic tasks, use headphones. You'll be inspired to move or dance as a result.
As a family, go for a dog walk.
How can I maintain an active routine?

The hardest aspect of starting a fitness regimen is keeping it up. But staying active may be made simpler with a few tips.

Maintain energy with meals
Eat a little snack, for instance, before working out to keep your energy levels up. However, nothing too hefty. excellent pre-workout snacks consist of:

stale food
banana
snack mix
a power bar
Crackers with peanut butter
adequate sleep
Sleep well the night before exercising as well. When you're groggy or worn out, working out is more difficult. Get a workout/accountability companion as well. This person inspires you to achieve your fitness objectives.

When you can, have fun.
Finally, pick exercises you love doing. Take a dancing class if you detest routine aerobics programs. Having fun makes staying active simpler.

The Value of Exercise and Weight Loss

Being overweight not only makes you feel uncomfortable, but it may also be harmful to your health. The Centers for Disease Control and Prevention (CDC) reports that obesity rates in the US have increased dramatically in recent years. By having a body mass index (BMI) of 30 or greater, obesity is characterized as affecting more than one-third of American people as of 2010. The formula for calculating body mass is weight in pounds divided by height in inches squared, and the result is then multiplied by 703 (weight (lb) / [height (in)] 2 x 703). You may determine your body mass by carrying out the following three steps:

Add 703 to your weight in pounds.
Determine your height in square inches.
Subtract the result of step 1 from the result of step 3, then multiply the result by 1.
Numerous major health issues, including heart disease, diabetes, stroke, and several forms of cancer, can be brought on by obesity.

Limiting the number of calories consumed through food is one strategy that might assist someone in losing weight. The alternative is to increase calorie burn through exercise.

advantages of exercise against diet
A healthier diet and regular exercise are both better for weight loss than calorie restriction alone. Certain illnesses' consequences can be avoided or even reversed by exercise. Exercise reduces cholesterol and blood pressure, which may help to stave against a heart attack.

Additionally, exercising reduces your chance of getting some malignancies, like colon and breast cancer. Exercise is also known to support feelings of confidence and well-being, perhaps reducing anxiety and depressive symptoms.

Exercise aids in weight reduction and weight maintenance. Exercise can boost metabolism, which is the number of calories you burn each day. Lean body mass may be maintained and increased, which also contributes to a daily calorie burn rise.

How Much Exercise Is Required to Lose Weight?
It is advised that you engage in some type of aerobic exercise at least three times a week for a minimum of 20 minutes per session if you want to benefit from exercise's health benefits. If you want to genuinely reduce weight, it's best to exercise for longer than 20 minutes. A daily regimen of just 15 minutes of moderate activity, such as walking a mile, can result in a 100-calorie calorie burn (provided you don't eat too many calories afterward). Ten pounds may be lost by burning 700 calories each week. of a year's worth of weight reduction.

What Are a Few Illustrations of the Various Exercise Forms?
What you select to exercise for weight reduction is less important than whether or not you do it. For this reason, experts advise choosing exercises you love to maintain a regular schedule.

Aerobic
Whatever fitness regimen you choose to follow should contain some sort of aerobic or cardiovascular activity. Exercises that are aerobic increase heart rate and blood circulation. Aerobic exercises include cycling, swimming, dancing, walking, and running. You can exercise with a fitness machine like a stair stepper, elliptical, or treadmill.

Strength Training
Gaining muscle when exercising with weights has several benefits, including helping you lose fat. In turn, muscle burns calories. What a positive feedback cycle! All main muscle groups should be worked out three times each week, according to experts. This comprises
biceps
calves
chest
forearms
hamstrings
quads
shoulders
traps
triceps

Yoga
According to a recent study by experts at the Fred Hutchinson Cancer Research Center, yoga is not as rigorous as other forms of exercise, but it can still aid in weight loss in other ways. According to the study, those

who practice yoga are less likely to be obese because they are more conscious of what they consume.

Making Exercise a Part of Your Lifestyle
More important than whether or not you exercise in a particular session is the overall quantity of activity you get in a day. Because of this, even little adjustments to your everyday routine can have a significant impact on your waistline.

Following a healthy lifestyle includes the following:

while running errands, riding your bike, or strolling to work
choosing to use the stairs rather than the elevator
parked further away and then completing the remaining distance on foot
The number of calories that different activities burn
To maintain his usual weight, the typical adult guy who doesn't exercise needs about 2,200 calories per day. To maintain her weight, a female needs about 1,800 calories daily.

The common activities on the list below, along with an estimate of how many calories they burn per hour:

240 to 300
cycling, dance, or vigorous exercise

370 to 460

walking (at a nine-minute-mile pace) or swimming, or playing football

580 to 730
racquetball, skiing, or running (at a seven-minute-mile pace)

740 to 920
Read More
Before Beginning an Exercise Program
Before beginning a new fitness regimen, especially if you want to engage in severe activity, see your doctor. This is particularly crucial if you have:

heart condition
lung condition
diabetes
renal illness
arthritis
Before beginning a new exercise program, people who have been very inactive lately, are overweight or have recently quit smoking should also consult their doctors.

It's crucial to pay attention to your body's cues when you initially begin a new fitness regimen. You should exert more effort so that your level of fitness increases. However, straining oneself beyond your limits might lead to harm. If you begin to feel discomfort or become breathless, stop exercising.

Chapter 3

## Basic Measures To Combat Obesity

You must concentrate on your mental health in addition to eating the appropriate foods and exercising regularly if you want to reduce weight. This is due to the fact that if you don't adopt the right mentality, your efforts to lose weight will be unsuccessful. Here are seven weight-loss suggestions.

1. Develop a philosophy of healthy living.

Weight management is more about living a healthy lifestyle than it is about having a weight-loss attitude. Put in place healthy living habits and try not to focus too much on your weight reduction. Instead, focus on getting enough exercise and eating the right foods. Living a satisfying life and taking care of your mental health are also essential components of healthy living. Until your head is in the right place, you won't be in the proper frame of mind to choose the right foods.

2. Make the choice to be joyful despite your current situation.

Some people make the decision that they won't be happy unless they lose a specific amount of weight or for some other reason. In other words, people need a license in order to be satisfied. The catch-22 is that having poor self-esteem will prevent you from controlling your weight. Your happiness is all your responsibility. Being the person you were meant to be will go a long way toward achieving happiness, and once you do, achieving your ideal weight will be simpler. You are responsible for choosing your own life's work.

3. Be genuine.

Be the finest version of yourself rather than a carbon duplicate of someone else since no one else is like you. It is preferable to cultivate your own unique qualities and talents rather than feeling envious of others who are brilliant in other areas. Instead of keeping or hoarding your abilities for yourself, you should share them with others so that others can profit from them. When it comes to weight reduction, it is useless to strive to develop a model-like figure if your body type is different.

4. Don't assess yourself against others.

Let everyone else finish their races before you focus on your own. People with low self-esteem typically make unfavorable comparisons to other people. It's true that individuals often date their self-esteem. They attract difficulties from those who share their experiences. Accept yourself as you are, and don't take it personally if others don't like you for who you are. Give it all you've got!

5. Don't pay attention to the commercials

Every available strategy will be used by marketers to grab your attention. Part of it is making you feel horrible about who you are. You can actually see why some ladies experience a decline in self-esteem when you watch some of the adverts. Be aware that there are many more people who tried their hardest but were unsuccessful for every individual who appears in those testimonies, as it is stated in the majority of commercials, "Results are not normal." Success stories that you read are usually exaggerated.

6. Skip the "before and after" commercials.

The before and after adverts are not worth your time. Only your own before and after photos should cause you concern. It's never appealing to see the before photo. You have no notion what happened to get the visually appealing outcome of the after shot.

7. everyday modest adjustments

Make gradual dietary changes to give your body time to adapt to a new routine, whether it's a change in what you eat or how you exercise. By implementing simple, attainable adjustments, cultivate good habits. Even if everything will take time, it is better to try to do too much too fast and then give up than to wait until the last minute. Keep in mind that nothing important has ever been produced in a day, even Rome.

8. Don't give up.

It might be demotivating if you are not making much progress. Keep trying; if you follow your healthy living plan, you will at least be assured that you are behaving morally. By focusing on your tasks, you may distract yourself from your worries. No matter what, appreciate every moment of life.

9. adopt new pastimes and activities

This is important for your wellbeing because if you are not in the right frame of mind, trying to manage your weight will not be successful. Are you familiar with the term "comfort eating"? Through interaction with people while playing a sport, you can widen your circle of friends and acquaintances. Sport participation surely contributes to weight management and mental stability maintenance. No matter how unfit you are, you may still take part in a number of sports. A little block walk is preferable to doing nothing except sitting on the couch. The key is to develop a habit of exercising.

10. Recognize that there are no secret formulae.

There is no trick to attaining the body you want. There isn't a quick answer or an easy remedy for losing weight. You must decide if the effort and cost were justified. There is a correct weight for every body type. Therefore, you must decide which body shape suits your weight the most.

 To be sure you are healthy enough to start an exercise regimen, check with your doctor first. Finding methods to include physical exercise into your day is the simplest approach to start exercising:

(1) Take the stairs rather than the elevator.

(2) At the grocery shop, park far from the front door.

(3) Sit on an exercise ball while working to build back and core strength.

(4) Take a stroll after work or after lunch.

(5) Exercise while watching TV by using hand weights or resistance bands.

(6) Play some music and start dancing.

(7) Be more active to reduce weight
It's time to begin exercising if your doctor advises you to reduce weight. You'll quickly discover that regular exercise has many advantages and is well worth the effort. Follow this straightforward advice to begin exercising:

Begin gradually.

If it's been a while since you've exercised, ease into your new workout routine and give your body some time to become used to it.

Choose a task you enjoy.
Enjoy the view while you bike or stroll through a local park. As you work out on an elliptical machine, listen to podcasts.

Work out with a friend.
Being social might help you stay motivated to work out more.

Remain hydrated.
Water is important to consume before, during  and after exercise.

Occasionally switch up your training regimen.
The diversity of physical activities you engage in keeps you engaged and keeps boredom at bay.

Put on a fitness monitor.
You may establish objectives using fitness trackers and health apps. Monitoring your development can inspire you.

What level of workout is required?
You engage in strength training at least twice per week, flexibility, and stretching activities, as well as at least 150 minutes of moderate cardiovascular activity each week. Focus on workouts that are easy on your joints if you

are overweight, such as walking, swimming, or water exercises.

If 150 minutes of exercise a week sounds overwhelming, divide your workout into smaller segments. Your objective should be to exercise for 30 minutes each day, five days a week. However, you are not required to do your 30-minute workout all at once. You may exercise for only 10 minutes at a time and still get results.

If you ever have chest discomfort, shortness of breath, nausea, pain in the neck or jaw, or any type of muscle or joint pain when exercising, stop immediately.

Celebrate your achievement.
Having a motivational factor to be active makes it simpler to incorporate exercise into your daily life. Identify strategies to recognize your weight loss accomplishments. After you accomplish a goal, get new exercise equipment. Or, once you drop five pounds, treat yourself to a massage. Just watch out that your incentives don't conflict with your objectives.

Chapter 4

Medication

People who have a BMI between 25 and 30 are considered to be overweight. Obesity is defined as having a BMI of 30 or greater. You can calculate your BMI NIH external link to learn if you are overweight, have obesity, or have severe obesity, which may increase your risk of health problems. Your healthcare professional can assess the risk caused by your weight.

If you are struggling with your weight, a healthy eating plan and regular physical activity may help you lose weight and keep it off over the long term. If these lifestyle changes are not enough to help you lose weight or maintain your weight loss, your healthcare professional may prescribe medications as part of your weight-control program.

How common are overweight and obesity?
Obesity is a chronic disease that affects more than 4 in 10 adults in the United States, and nearly 1 in 10 Americans have severe obesity.

How do weight management medications work?
Prescription medications to treat overweight and obesity work in different ways. For example, some medications may help you feel less hungry or full sooner. Other medications may make it harder for your body to absorb fat from the foods you eat.

Who might benefit from weight management medications?

Weight management medications are meant to help people who have health problems related to being overweight or obese. Healthcare professionals use BMI to help decide whether you might benefit from weight management medications. Your health care professional may prescribe a medication to treat your overweight or obesity if you are an adult with

a BMI of 30 or greater a BMI of 27 or greater, and you have weight-related health problems such as high blood pressure NIH external link or type 2 diabetes
Weight management medications aren't for everyone with a high BMI. If you are overweight or have obesity, you might be able to lose weight with a lifestyle program that changes your behaviors and improves your eating and physical activity habits. A lifestyle program may also address other things that cause you to gain weight, such as eating triggers and not getting enough sleep.

Can children or teenagers take weight management medications?

Most of the weight management medications approved by the U.S. Food and Drug Administration External link (FDA) are for adults only. Two prescription medications, orlistat NIH external link (Xenical)2 and liraglutide (Saxenda),3 are approved by the FDA for children ages 12 and older. A third prescription medication, bremelanotide (IMCIVREE),4 is approved by the FDA

for children ages 6 years and older who have rare
genetic disorders causing obesity.

Can medications replace physical activity and healthy
eating habits as a way to lose weight?
Medications don't replace physical activity or healthy
eating habits as a way to lose weight. Studies show that
weight management medications work best when
combined with a lifestyle program. Ask your healthcare
professional about lifestyle treatment programs for
weight management that will work for you.

Two women walking down a paved road with earbuds in
their ears.
Weight management medications don't replace physical
activity and healthy eating habits.
What are the benefits of using prescription medications
to lose weight?
When combined with behavior changes, including
healthy eating and increased physical activity,
prescription medications help some people lose weight
and maintain weight loss. On average, after 1 year,
people who take prescription medications as part of a
lifestyle program lose 3% to 12% more of their starting
body weight than people in a lifestyle program who do
not take medication.

Research shows that some people taking prescription
weight management medications lose 10% or more of
their starting weight.5,6 Results vary by medication and
by a person.

Weight loss of 5% to 10% of your starting body weight may help improve your health by lowering blood sugar, blood pressure, and triglyceride levels. Losing weight also can improve some other health problems related to being overweight and obesity, such as joint pain and sleep apnea. Most weight loss takes place within the first 6 months of starting the medication.

What are the concerns about using prescription medications to lose weight?
Experts are concerned that, in some cases, the side effects of prescription medications that treat overweight and obesity may outweigh the benefits. For this reason, never take weight management medication only to improve the way you look. In the past, some weight management medications were linked to serious health problems, and they were removed from U.S. markets.

Possible side effects vary by medication and how it acts on your body. Most side effects are mild and most often improve if you continue to take the medication. Rarely, serious side effects can occur.

Tips for taking weight management medication
Follow your healthcare professional's instructions about weight management medications.
Buy your medication from a pharmacy or online distributor approved by your healthcare professional.
Only take weight management medication to support your healthy eating and physical activity program.

Know the side effects and warnings before taking any medication.

If you are not losing weight after 12 weeks on the full dose of your medication, ask your healthcare professional whether you should stop taking it.

Talk with your health care professional about any other medications you are taking, including supplements and vitamins, when considering weight management medications.

Never take weight management medications during pregnancy or if you are planning a pregnancy.

Which weight management medication might work for me?

Choosing a medication to treat overweight or obesity is a decision between you and your health care professional. Important factors to consider include

If you have lost enough weight to improve your health and are not experiencing serious side effects, your healthcare professional may advise you to stay on the medication indefinitely. If you do not lose at least 5% of your starting weight after 12 weeks on the full dose of your medication, your healthcare professional will probably advise you to stop taking it. Your healthcare professional may also

change your treatment plan or consider using a different weight management medication
have you tried different lifestyles, physical activity, or eating programs

change your other medications that might be causing weight gain
refer you to a bariatric surgeon to see if weight-loss (bariatric) surgery  might be an option for you
Because obesity is a chronic disease, you may need to continue your new eating and physical activity habits and other behaviors for years—or even a lifetime—to improve your health and maintain a healthier weight.

Will I regain some weight after I stop taking weight management medication?
You probably will regain some weight after you stop taking weight management medication. Developing and maintaining healthy eating habits and increasing physical activity may help you regain less weight or keep it off.

What medications are available to treat overweight and obesity?
The table below lists prescription drugs approved by the FDA for weight loss. The FDA has approved five of these drugs—orlistat (Xenical, Alli), phentermine-topiramate (Qsymia), naltrexone-bupropion (Contrave), liraglutide (Saxenda), and semaglutide (Wegovy)—for long-term use. A sixth approved drug, bremelanotide (IMCIVREE), is limited to people who have been diagnosed with one of three specific rare genetic disorders, which must be confirmed by genetic testing. You can keep taking these medications as long as you are benefiting from treatment and not experiencing serious side effects.

Some weight management medications that curb appetite are approved by the FDA for short-term use only, for up to 12 weeks. Although some healthcare professionals prescribe them for longer periods, not many research studies have looked at how safe and effective they are for long-term use.

Never take weight management medications if you are pregnant. If you are planning to get pregnant, you should also avoid these medications, as some of them may harm the fetus.

Prescription medications approved to treat overweight and obesity
Weight Management Medication   Approved For   How It Works   Common Side Effects   Warnings
orlistat NIH external link (Xenical)

Available in lower doses without a prescription (Alli) for Adults and children ages 12 and older   Works in your gut to reduce the amount of fat your body absorbs from the food you eat
diarrhea
gas
leakage of oily stools
stomach pain
Rare cases of severe liver injury have been reported
Avoid taking with cyclosporine NIH external link

Take a multivitamin pill daily to make sure you get enough of certain vitamins that your body may not absorb from the food you eat
phentermine-topiramate NIH external link (Qsymia)
Adults
A mix of two medications: phentermine, which lessens your appetite, and topiramate, which is used to treat seizures or migraine headaches
May make you less hungry or feel full sooner
constipation
dizziness
dry mouth
taste changes, especially with carbonated beverages
tingling of your hands and feet
trouble sleeping
Do not use it if you have glaucoma or hyperthyroidism
Tell your healthcare professional if you have had a heart attack or stroke, abnormal heart rhythm, kidney disease, or mood problems
MAY LEAD TO BIRTH DEFECTS.DO NOT TAKE PHENTERMINE-TOPIRAMATE IF YOU ARE PREGNANT OR ARE PLANNING A PREGNANCY
Do not take it if you are breastfeeding
naltrexone-bupropion NIH external link (Contrave)
Adults
A mix of two medications: naltrexone, which is used to treat alcohol and drug dependence, and bupropion, which is used to treat depression or help people quit smoking
May make you feel less hungry or full sooner
constipation

diarrhea
dizziness
dry mouth
headache
increased blood pressure
increased heart rate
insomnia
liver damage
nausea
vomiting
Do not use if you have uncontrolled high blood pressure,
seizures, or a history of anorexia or bulimia nervosa
Do not use if you are dependent on opioid pain
medications or are withdrawing from drugs or alcohol
Do not use it if you are taking bupropion (Wellbutrin,
Zyban)
MAY INCREASE SUICIDAL THOUGHTS OR ACTIONS
liraglutide NIH external link (Saxenda)

Given daily by injection, Adults and children ages 12
years and older
Mimics a hormone called glucagon-like peptide-1
(GLP-1) that targets areas of the brain that regulate
appetite and food intake
At a lower dose under a different name, Victoza, this
drug was FDA-approved to treat type 2 diabetes
nausea
diarrhea
constipation
abdominal pain
headache

increased heart rate
This may increase the chance of developing pancreatitis
Has been found to cause a rare type of thyroid tumor in
animals
semaglutide (Wegovy)

Given weekly by injection    Adults
Mimics a hormone called glucagon-like peptide-1
(GLP-1) that targets areas of the brain that regulate
appetite and food intake
Under different names and dosages, this drug was
FDA-approved to treat type 2 diabetes as an injectable
medication (Ozempic) and as an oral pill (Rybelsus)
nausea
diarrhea
vomiting
constipation
abdominal (stomach) pain
headache
fatigue
Do not use in combination with other
semaglutide-containing products, other GLP-1 receptor
agonists, or other products intended for weight loss,
including prescription drugs, over-the-counter drugs, or
herbal products
This may increase the chance of developing pancreatitis
Has been found to cause a rare type of thyroid tumor in
animals
setmelanotide (IMCIVREE)

Available by injection only People who have a BMI between 25 and 30 are considered to be overweight. Obesity is defined as having a BMI of 30 or greater. You can calculate your BMI NIH external link to learn if you are overweight, have obesity, or have severe obesity, which may increase your risk of health problems. Your healthcare professional can assess the risk caused by your weight.

If you are struggling with your weight, a healthy eating plan and regular physical activity may help you lose weight and keep it off over the long term. If these lifestyle changes are not enough to help you lose weight or maintain your weight loss, your healthcare professional may prescribe medications as part of your weight-control program.

How common are overweight and obesity?
Obesity is a chronic disease that affects more than 4 in 10 adults in the United States, and nearly 1 in 10 Americans have severe obesity.

How do weight management medications work?
Prescription medications to treat overweight and obesity work in different ways. For example, some medications may help you feel less hungry or full sooner. Other medications may make it harder for your body to absorb fat from the foods you eat.

Who might benefit from weight management medications?

Weight management medications are meant to help people who have health problems related to overweight or obese. Healthcare professionals use BMI to help decide whether you might benefit from weight management medications. Your health care professional may prescribe a medication to treat your overweight or obesity if you are an adult with a BMI of 30 or greater a BMI of 27 or greater, and you have weight-related health problems such as high blood pressure NIH external link or type 2 diabetes.

Weight management medications aren't for everyone with a high BMI. If you are overweight or have obesity, you might be able to lose weight with a lifestyle program that changes your behaviors and improves your eating and physical activity habits. A lifestyle program may also address other things that cause you to gain weight, such as eating triggers and not getting enough sleep.

Can children or teenagers take weight management medications?
Most of the weight management medications approved by the U.S. Food and Drug Administration External link (FDA) are for adults only. Two prescription medications, orlistat NIH external link (Xenical)2 and liraglutide (Saxenda),3 are approved by the FDA for children ages 12 and older. A third prescription medication, bremelanotide (IMCIVREE),4 is approved by the FDA for children ages 6 years and older who have rare genetic disorders causing obesity.

Can medications replace physical activity and healthy eating habits as a way to lose weight?

Medications don't replace physical activity or healthy eating habits as a way to lose weight. Studies show that weight management medications work best when combined with a lifestyle program. Ask your healthcare professional about lifestyle treatment programs for weight management that will work for you.

Two women walking down a paved road with earbuds in their ears.

Weight management medications don't replace physical activity and healthy eating habits.

What are the benefits of using prescription medications to lose weight?

When combined with behavior changes, including healthy eating and increased physical activity, prescription medications help some people lose weight and maintain weight loss. On average, after 1 year, people who take prescription medications as part of a lifestyle program lose 3% to 12% more of their starting body weight than people in a lifestyle program who do not take medication.

Research shows that some people taking prescription weight management medications lose 10% or more of their starting weight.5,6 Results vary by medication and by a person.

Weight loss of 5% to 10% of your starting body weight may help improve your health by lowering blood sugar blood pressure, and triglyceride levels. Losing weight also can improve some other health problems related to being overweight and obesity, such as joint pain and sleep apnea. Most weight loss takes place within the first 6 months of starting the medication.

What are the concerns about using prescription medications to lose weight?
Experts are concerned that, in some cases, the side effects of prescription medications that treat overweight and obesity may outweigh the benefits. For this reason, never take weight management medication only to improve the way you look. In the past, some weight management medications were linked to serious health problems, and they were removed from U.S. markets.

Possible side effects vary by medication and how it acts on your body. Most side effects are mild and most often improve if you continue to take the medication. Rarely, serious side effects can occur.

Tips for taking weight management medication
Follow your healthcare professional's instructions about weight management medications.
Buy your medication from a pharmacy or online distributor approved by your healthcare professional.
Only take weight management medication to support your healthy eating and physical activity program.
Know the side effects and warnings before taking any medication.

If you are not losing weight after 12 weeks on the full dose of your medication, ask your healthcare professional whether you should stop taking it.
Talk with your health care professional about any other medications you are taking, including supplements and vitamins, when considering weight management medications.
Never take weight management medications during pregnancy or if you are planning a pregnancy.

Which weight management medication might work for me?
Choosing a medication to treat overweight or obesity is a decision between you and your health care professional. Important factors to consider include

If you have lost enough weight to improve your health and are not experiencing serious side effects, your healthcare professional may advise you to stay on the medication indefinitely. If you do not lose at least 5% of your starting weight after 12 weeks on the full dose of your medication, your healthcare professional will probably advise you to stop taking it. Your healthcare professional may also

change your treatment plan or consider using a different weight management medication
have you tried different lifestyles, physical activity, or eating programs
change your other medications that might be causing weight gain

refer you to a bariatric surgeon to see if weight-loss (bariatric) surgery  might be an option for you
Because obesity is a chronic disease, you may need to continue your new eating and physical activity habits and other behaviors for years—or even a lifetime—to improve your health and maintain a healthier weight.

Will I regain some weight after I stop taking weight management medication?
You probably will regain some weight after you stop taking weight management medication. Developing and maintaining healthy eating habits and increasing physical activity may help you regain less weight or keep it off.

What medications are available to treat overweight and obesity?
The table below lists prescription drugs approved by the FDA for weight loss. The FDA has approved five of these drugs—orlistat (Xenical, Alli), phentermine-topiramate (Qsymia), naltrexone-bupropion (Contrave), liraglutide (Saxenda), and semaglutide (Wegovy)—for long-term use. A sixth approved drug, bremelanotide (IMCIVREE), is limited to people who have been diagnosed with one of three specific rare genetic disorders, which must be confirmed by genetic testing. You can keep taking these medications as long as you are benefiting from treatment and not experiencing serious side effects.

Some weight management medications that curb appetite are approved by the FDA for short-term use only, for up to 12 weeks. Although some healthcare professionals prescribe them for longer periods, not many research studies have looked at how safe and effective they are for long-term use.

Never take weight management medications if you are pregnant. If you are planning to get pregnant, you should also avoid these medications, as some of them may harm the fetus.

Prescription medications approved to treat overweight and obesity
Weight Management Medication    Approved For    How It Works    Common Side Effects    Warnings
orlistat NIH external link (Xenical)

Available in lower doses without a prescription (Alli) for Adults and children ages 12 and older    Works in your gut to reduce the amount of fat your body absorbs from the food you eat
diarrhea
gas
leakage of oily stools
stomach pain
Rare cases of severe liver injury have been reported
Avoid taking with cyclosporine NIH external link
Take a multivitamin pill daily to make sure you get enough of certain vitamins that your body may not absorb from the food you eat

phentermine-topiramate NIH external link (Qsymia)
Adults
A mix of two medications: phentermine, which lessens
your appetite, and topiramate, which is used to treat
seizures or migraine headaches
May make you less hungry or feel full sooner
constipation
dizziness
dry mouth
taste changes, especially with carbonated beverages
tingling of your hands and feet
trouble sleeping
Do not use it if you have glaucoma or hyperthyroidism
Tell your healthcare professional if you have had a heart
attack or stroke, abnormal heart rhythm, kidney disease,
or mood problems
MAY LEAD TO BIRTH DEFECTS.DO NOT TAKE
PHENTERMINE-TOPIRAMATE IF YOU ARE
PREGNANT OR ARE PLANNING A PREGNANCY
Do not take it if you are breastfeeding
naltrexone-bupropion NIH external link (Contrave)
Adults
A mix of two medications: naltrexone, which is used to
treat alcohol and drug dependence, and bupropion,
which is used to treat depression or help people quit
smoking
May make you feel less hungry or full sooner
constipation
diarrhea
dizziness
dry mouth

headache
increased blood pressure
increased heart rate
insomnia
liver damage
nausea
vomiting
Do not use if you have uncontrolled high blood pressure,
seizures, or a history of anorexia or bulimia nervosa
Do not use if you are dependent on opioid pain
medications or are withdrawing from drugs or alcohol
Do not use it if you are taking bupropion (Wellbutrin,
Zyban)
MAY INCREASE SUICIDAL THOUGHTS OR ACTIONS
liraglutide NIH external link (Saxenda)

Given daily by injection, Adults and children ages 12
years and older
Mimics a hormone called glucagon-like peptice-1
(GLP-1) that targets areas of the brain that regulate
appetite and food intake
At a lower dose under a different name, Victoza, this
drug was FDA-approved to treat type 2 diabetes
nausea
diarrhea
constipation
abdominal pain
headache
increased heart rate
This may increase the chance of developing pancreatitis

Has been found to cause a rare type of thyroid tumor in animals

semaglutide (Wegovy)7

Given weekly by injection    Adults

Mimics a hormone called glucagon-like peptide-1 (GLP-1) that targets areas of the brain that regulate appetite and food intake

Under different names and dosages, this drug was FDA-approved to treat type 2 diabetes as an injectable medication (Ozempic) and as an oral pill (Rybelsus)

nausea

diarrhea

vomiting

constipation

abdominal (stomach) pain

headache

fatigue

Do not use in combination with other semaglutide-containing products, other GLP-1 receptor agonists, or other products intended for weight loss, including prescription drugs, over-the-counter drugs, or herbal products

This may increase the chance of developing pancreatitis

Has been found to cause a rare type of thyroid tumor in animals

setmelanotide (IMCIVREE)

Available by injection only    People ages 6 years and older with obesity due to three specific rare genetic conditions only

May reduce appetite and increase the feeling of fullness
May increase resting metabolism (how the body burns calories)
Although it can help a person lose weight, it does not treat the genetic defects
injection site reaction
skin darkening
nausea
disturbance in sexual arousal
depression and suicidal ideation
risk of serious adverse reactions in neonates and infants with low birth weight, owing to the benzyl alcohol preservative
Only for people with any of these ultra-rare genetic diseases, confirmed by genetic testing
proopiomelanocortin (POMC) deficiency
proprotein convertase subtilisin/Kexin type 1 (PCSK1) deficiency
leptin receptor (LEPR) deficiency
Do not use it while pregnant or breastfeeding.
(Other medications that curb your desire to eat include)
phentermine
benzphetamine
diethylpropion
phendimetrazine

Adults
Increases chemicals in your brain to make you feel you are not hungry or that you are full
Note: FDA-approved only for short-term use—up to 12 weeks

dry mouth
constipation
difficulty sleeping
dizziness
feeling nervous
feeling restless
headache
raised blood pressure
increased heart rate
Do not use if you have heart disease, uncontrolled high
blood pressure, hyperthyroidism, or glaucoma
Tell your healthcare professional if you have severe
anxiety or other mental health problems
How do healthcare professionals use prescription
medications "off-label" to treat overweight and obesity?
Sometimes health care professionals use medications in
a way that's different from what the FDA has approved.
That's called "off-label" use. By choosing an off-label
medication to treat overweight and obesity, your
healthcare professional may prescribe

a drug approved for treating a different medical problem
two or more drugs at the same time
a drug for a longer period than approved by the FDA
You should feel comfortable asking whether your
healthcare professional is prescribing a medication that
is not approved for treating overweight and obesity.
Before using a medication, learn all you need to know
about it.

What other medications for weight loss may be available in the future?
Researchers are currently studying several new medications and combinations of medications in animals and people. Researchers are working to identify safer and more effective medications to help people who are overweight or have obesity lose weight and maintain a healthy weight for a long time.

Future drugs may use new strategies, such as
regulating several gut hormones at the same time
targeting specific genes that cause obesity
allowing people to lose body fat without losing muscle during weight loss
changing bacteria in the gut to control weight
Clinical Trials for Prescription Medications to Treat Overweight and Obesity
The NIDDK conducts and supports clinical trials in many diseases and conditions, including overweight and obesity. The trials look to find new ways to prevent, detect, or treat disease and improve quality of life.

What are clinical trials for prescription medications to treat overweight and obesity?
Clinical trials—and other types of clinical studies NIH external link—are part of medical research and involve people like you. When you volunteer to take part in a clinical study, you help healthcare professionals and researchers learn more about the disease and improve health care for people in the future.

Researchers are studying many aspects of prescription medications to treat overweight or obesity NIH external link, such as

the effect of the FDA-approved medication liraglutide (Saxenda, Victoza) on weight loss and gastric functions (stomach emptying effect) in people who are overweight or have obesity
adolescents and young adults who don't achieve expected weight loss or who still have severe obesity after undergoing weight-loss surgery
patients who have obesity and binge-eating disorder
women who are overweight or have obesity and polycystic ovary syndrome NIH external link
Find out if clinical studies are right for your NIH external link.

People ages 6 years and older with obesity due to three specific rare genetic conditions only
May reduce appetite and increase the feeling of fullness
May increase resting metabolism (how the body burns calories)
Although it can help a person lose weight, it does not treat the genetic defects
injection site reaction
skin darkening
nausea
disturbance in sexual arousal
depression and suicidal ideation
risk of serious adverse reactions in neonates and infants with low birth weight, owing to the benzyl alcohol preservative

Only for people with any of these ultra-rare genetic
diseases, confirmed by genetic testing
proopiomelanocortin (POMC) deficiency
proprotein convertase subtilisin/Kexin type 1 (PCSK1)
deficiency
leptin receptor (LEPR) deficiency
Do not use it while pregnant or breastfeeding.
(Other medications that curb your desire to eat include)
phentermine
benzphetamine
diethylpropion
phendimetrazine
Adults
Increases chemicals in your brain to make you feel you
are not hungry or that you are full
Note: FDA-approved only for short-term use—up to 12
weeks
dry mouth
constipation
difficulty sleeping
dizziness
feeling nervous
feeling restless
headache
raised blood pressure
increased heart rate

Do not use if you have heart disease, uncontrolled high
blood pressure, hyperthyroidism, or glaucoma
Tell your healthcare professional if you have severe
anxiety or other mental health problems

How do healthcare professionals use prescription medications "off-label" to treat overweight and obesity?
Sometimes health care professionals use medications in a way that's different from what the FDA has approved. That's called "off-label" use. By choosing an off-label medication to treat overweight and obesity, your healthcare professional may prescribe a drug approved for treating a different medical problem
two or more drugs at the same time
a drug for a longer time than approved by the FDA
You should feel comfortable asking whether your healthcare professional is prescribing a medication that is not approved for treating overweight and obesity. Before using a medication, learn all you need to know about it.

What other medications for weight loss may be available in the future?
Researchers are currently studying several new medications and combinations of medications in animals and people. Researchers are working to identify safer and more effective medications to help people who are overweight or have obesity lose weight and maintain a healthy weight for a long time.

Future drugs may use new strategies, such as

regulating several gut hormones at the same time
targeting specific genes that cause obesity
allowing people to lose body fat without losing muscle during weight loss

changing bacteria in the gut to control weight
Clinical Trials for Prescription Medications to Treat
Overweight and Obesity
The NIDDK conducts and supports clinical trials in many
diseases and conditions, including overweight and
obesity. The trials look to find new ways to prevent,
detect, or treat disease and improve quality of life.

What are clinical trials for prescription medications to
treat overweight and obesity?
Clinical trials—and other types of clinical studies NIH
external link—are part of medical research and involve
people like you. When you volunteer to take part in a
clinical study, you help healthcare professionals and
researchers learn more about the disease and improve
health care for people in the future.

Researchers are studying many aspects of prescription
medications to treat overweight or obesity NIH external
link, such as

the effect of the FDA-approved medication liraglutide
(Saxenda, Victoza) on weight loss and gastric functions
(stomach emptying effect) in people who are overweight
or have obesity
adolescents and young adults who don't achieve
expected weight loss or who still have severe obesity
after undergoing weight-loss surgery
patients who have obesity and binge-eating disorder
women who are overweight or have obesity and
polycystic ovary syndrome NIH external link

Find out if clinical studies are right for your NIH external link.

Chapter 5

Weight Loss Diet Chart Plan

As the name suggests, a low-fat diet restricts the intake of fat to no more than around one-third of the daily caloric intake. It has minimal fat, especially saturated fats and cholesterol, which raise blood cholesterol levels and increase the risk of a heart attack.

This kind of weight-loss diet plan emphasizes foods with healthy grains, fruits, and vegetables. By providing 20 to 30% of daily total calories as fat, it promotes weight loss and the treatment of several disorders. A normal low-fat diet provides the body with plenty of veggies, proteins, and relatively little fat.

While some dietary fat is necessary for optimal health, providing energy and fat-soluble vitamins like A, D, E, and K, it shouldn't be completely removed. According to studies, the appropriate types of lipids might really aid n weight loss. As a result, cutting back on bad fats and increasing consumption of healthy fats are the main goals of a healthy diet plan for obesity.

Diets low in fat have been encouraged to prevent heart disease. It has been demonstrated that reducing fat intake from 35–40% of total calories to 15-20% of total calories will lower total and LDL cholesterol by 10–20%; however, the majority of this reduction is attributable to a drop in saturated fat intake.

We design an Indian diet plan for those who are obese. Start eating the foods specified for breakfast, lunch, and supper if you decide to stick to this diet plan

Diet plan for obesity patient Sunday

Breakfast (8:00-8:30AM)   3 egg whites + 1 toasted brown bread + 1/2 cup low fat milk (no sugar)
Mid-Meal (11:00-11:30AM)   1 cup papaya
Lunch (2:00-2:30PM)   1 cup arhar dal + 1 chapatti + 1/2 cup low fat curd + salad
Evening (4:00-4:30 PM)   1 cup vegetable soup
Dinner (8:00-8:30 PM)   1 cup pumpkin + 1 chapatti + salad
Monday
Breakfast (8:00-8:30 AM)   1 onion stuffed chapatti + 1/2 cup low-fat curd
Mid-Meal (11:00-11:30 AM)   1 cup coconut water
Lunch (2:00-2:30 PM)   1 cup moong dal/ chicken curry + 1 chapatti + salad
Evening (4:00-4:30 PM)   1 cup pomegranate
Dinner (8:00-8:30 PM)   1 cup of beans + 1 chapatti + salad
Tuesday
Breakfast (8:00-8:30 AM)   2 besan cheela + 1/2 cup low-fat curd
Mid-Meal (11:00-11:30 AM)   1 apple
Lunch (2:00-2:30PM)   1 cup masoor dal + 1 chapatti + 1/2 up low fat curd + salad
Evening (4:00-4:30 PM)   1 cup tomato soup

Dinner (8:00-8:30 PM)    1 cup carrot peas vegetable +1 chapatti + salad

Wednesday

Breakfast (8:00-8:30 AM)    1 cup vegetable brown bread upma + 1/2 cup low-fat milk (no sugar)

Mid-Meal (11:00-11:30 AM)    1 cup musk melon

Lunch (2:00-2:30 PM)    1 cup rajma curry + 1 chapatti + salad

Evening (4:00-4:30 PM)    1 cup vegetable soup

Dinner (8:00-8:30 PM)    1 cup parwal vegetable + 1 chapatti + salad

Thursday

Breakfast (8:00-8:30 AM)    1 cucumber hung curd sandwich + 1/2 tsp green chutney + 1 orange

Mid-Meal (11:00-11:30 AM)    1 cup buttermilk

Lunch (2:00-2:30 PM)    1 cup white chana/ fish curry + 1 chapatti + salad

Evening (4:00-4:30 PM)    1 cup low-fat milk (no sugar)

Dinner (8:00-8:30 PM)    1 cup cauliflower vegetable + 1 chapatti + salad

Friday

Breakfast (8:00-8:30 AM)    1 cup vegetable poha + 1 cup low-fat curd

Mid-Meal (11:00-11:30 AM)    1 cup watermelon

Lunch (2:00-2:30 PM)    1 cup chana dal + 1 chapatti + salad

Evening (4:00-4:30 PM)    1 cup sprouts salad

Dinner (8:00-8:30 PM)    1 cup tienda vegetable + 1 chapatti + salad

Saturday

Breakfast (8:00-8:30 AM)    1 cup low-fat milk with oats + 3-4 strawberries
Mid-Meal (11:00-11:30 AM)    1 cup coconut water
Lunch (2:00-2:30PM)    1 cup soybean curry + 1 chapatti + 1/2 cup low fat curd + salad
Evening (4:00-4:30 PM)    1 cup fruit salad
Dinner (8:00-8:30 PM)    1 cup ghia vegetable + 1 chapatti + salad
Do's And Dont While following Diet Plan for Obesity
Try to avoid these food items if you are following an obesity diet plan:

Rely on soft drinks, sweetened cereals, cookies and cakes, donuts and pastries, chips, and confectionery to get you through the day.

Don't skip meals. This will tempt you to snack and DO NOT snack between meals
Avoid eating quickly. Sit and chew each bite. Try using chopsticks!

Don't food shop when you're hungry.
Don't eat more than two or three pieces of fruit per day.
Add these food items if your diet chart if you are following an obesity diet plan :

Eat more vegetables ,add them to every meal.

Drink plenty of water - you can become hungry when thirsty.
Try eating off smaller plates to eat smaller portions

Exercise between 30 minutes to one hour each day with moderate exercise - brisk walking, team sport, cycling, or swimming.

Be mindful of what you put in your mouth and your shopping trolley.

Food Items You Can Easily Consume In Obesity Diet Plan

Choose minimally processed, whole foods:

Whole grains (whole wheat, steel-cut oats, brown rice, quinoa)

Vegetables (a colorful variety-not potatoes)

Whole fruits (not fruit juices)

Nuts, seeds, beans, and other healthful sources of protein (fish and poultry)

Plant oils (olive and other vegetable oils)

Drink water or other beverages that are naturally calorie-free

The components of the optimum diet chart may be discussed in great detail. One's dietary needs, however, vary depending on many things. It could vary based on gender, for instance, as male and female nutritional needs are different.

Geographical factors may also be at play because the cuisines of North and South India differ significantly. Since a vegetarian or vegan consumes food quite differently from a non-vegetarian, meal choices become important in this situation.

However, we have created a diet strategy that is great for losing weight while eating Indian food. This sample 7-day diet plan, commonly known as a 1200-calorie diet plan, is for educational purposes only and should not be used by anybody without first visiting a nutritionist.

Add the following nutrients to your diet plan a result:

1. Dietary Plan for Carbohydrates
The majority of the daily calories you need should come from carbohydrates because they are the body's primary energy source. However, it's crucial to pick the proper kind of carbohydrates. Simple carbohydrates, such as bread, biscuits, white rice, and wheat flour, are unhealthy because they are too sweet.

As opposed to simple carbohydrates, choose complex carbs since they are higher in fiber and include more nutrients. This is because complex carbohydrates high in fiber take longer to digest and make you feel fuller for longer, making them the greatest choice for weight management.

Oats, brown rice, and millets like ragi are all excellent sources of complex carbohydrates.

2. Dietary Proteins
The majority of Indians don't get enough protein each day. This is problematic since the body needs proteins to pump blood and develop and repair tissue, muscles, cartilage, and skin. Hence. A diet rich in protein can also

aid in weight loss since it promotes muscle growth, which burns more calories than fat.

For instance, you should include protein in your diet in the form of entire dals, paneer, chana, milk, leafy greens, eggs, white meat, or sprouts, making up roughly 30% of your total calories. Every meal has to include one serving of protein.

protein-rich foods for the ideal Indian diet

3. Diet for Fats
Although they have a poor image, fats are an important dietary category because they help the body create hormones, store vitamins, and provide us energy. One-fifth or 20% of your diet, according to experts, should be made up of polyunsaturated, monounsaturated, and Omega-3 fatty acids.

The best method to ingest fats, for instance, is to use a variety of oils for different meals, such as olive oil, rice bran oil, mustard oil, soya bean, sesame, sunflower, and groundnut oil, along with moderate amounts of butter and ghee. But for a well-balanced Indian diet plan, you must eliminate trans fats, which are present in fried foods.

4. Nutrients and vitamins
Food menu For the body to operate properly and to promote metabolism, neuron and muscle function, bone maintenance, and cell creation, vitamins A, E, B12, and

D, calcium, and iron are necessary. Minerals are also present in foods like nuts, oilseeds, fruits, and green leafy vegetables because they are generally sourced from plants, meat, and fish.

Nutritionists and experts advise eating 100 grams of fruits and 100 grams of vegetables each day.

5. Meal Substitutions in the Indian Weight Loss Diet
Replace the bad items in your Indian Diet plan with their better equivalents for one of the simplest methods to eat healthily.

For instance, air-popped popcorn instead of potato chips might satisfy your urge for a snack to nibble on. Therefore, it would be wonderful if you looked into some healthy meal replacement choices that you may attempt in the future.

These routines will assist you in maintaining your health together with a balanced meal plan for weight loss:

Instead of three large meals, try having three smaller meals and a few snack breaks throughout the day in controlled portions. By spreading out your meals at regular intervals, you can avoid bloating and acid reflux while also avoiding hunger pangs. So, give up eating junk food by incorporating healthier snack options into your Indian diet plan.

Eat dinner earlier

Other societies around the world tend to eat cinner later than Indians do. After dinner, metabolism slows down, which can result in weight gain. By 8 p.m., experts advise eating your final meal of the day.

Drink a lot of water:
How can increasing your water intake assist in weight loss? First off, there are no calories in it. A glass of water might also help quell hunger cravings. To lose weight, drink six to eight glasses of water every day. You can also discover a list of beverages that can aid in weight loss here.

Eat plenty of fiber
Fiber helps with digestion and heart health, so an individual needs at least 15 gm of it daily. Some excellent sources of fiber include apples, broccoli, lentils, flax seeds, and lentils.